Table of content

I0086196

Introduction

Introduction

In front of you is the educational workbook:
"Your Guide to a Positive Life.
Workbook VI: Memory and Concentration - Exercises".
This is another dose of knowledge that will allow you to discover the power that flows from your interior.

Our collaborative workbook will allow you to:
• increase concentration,
• activate the natural mechanism of development,
• increase your physical and intellectual activity,
• improve short-term and long-term memory,
• develop mental processes: the ability to clearly formulate thoughts and to think abstractly,

Thanks to simple techniques for activating your brain, you will become more open to the world and the people around you.

Your memory and concentration will still be in great shape!

Your time is now. Get control over your:
life - health - relationships - dreams

Remember, you are doing this for you!

I wish you the best of luck in discovering your true self!
Kasia Dorosz

CHALLENGE YOUR MIND, NO MATTER WHAT YOUR AGE!

Read, write, solve crosswords, learn languages,
play board games.

An observational study published on May 30, 2018 by JAMA Psychiatry demonstrated that engaging in stimulating intellectual activities, even at a mature age, can reduce the chances of dementia.

Researchers have observed over 15,000 70-year-old Chinese men and women for seven years. They carried out an annual assessment of health habits and lifestyle, including various recreational activities. The study showed that people who challenged their brains daily, such as by playing board games, reading and even betting on races, were 29% less likely to be diagnosed with dementia than people who chose other activities: recreational (watching television, shopping) or socialization.

What is good for Your heart
is also good for Your mind.

A French study published on August 21, 2018 in The Journal of the American Medical Association suggests that the more steps you take to improve cardiovascular health, the lower your risk of developing dementia. Scientists have evaluated health and lifestyle data for over 6 thousand men free from dementia and men with heart disease at the age of 70. They wanted to see what would happen when they started using the 7 steps recommended by the American Heart Association, i.e. not smoking; weight control; regular physical activity; eating a healthy diet and maintaining healthy blood pressure, cholesterol and blood sugar levels.

5-MINUTE EXERCISES FOR BETTER HEALTH

Adopting a new health routine can be difficult. Performing short tasks that contribute to health may be easier to achieve.
Do you know what you should do?
• Exercise everyday
• Give up unhealthy food
• Ensure a good night´s sleep
• Carefully monitor every aspect of your health

It is a great commitment that seems like a serious undertaking if you have never done it before. However, putting off a healthy life-style for later increases the risk of developing chronic diseases.

Rather than procrastinate, focus on small tasks that will not overwhelm you. Try to exercise from time to time, even for 5 minutes.

„Doing something, even small bursts of activity, such as climbing a few stairs or starting a day with a few minutes of physical exercise, leads to measurable health benefits. Nobody should think that the effort of moving is not enough.„

- Dr. Aaron Baggish, director of the Cardiovascular Performance Program at the Harvard-Massachusetts General Hospital

Exercise more!
If planning a long workout is difficult, put a simple five-minute workout on your to-do list: walk in place, do some lifts or sit-ups.

WRITING MESSAGES IS MORE POWERFUL THAN YOU THINK

Writing thank-you messages is not just good manners. This activity may have a strong psychological effect on both the sender and recipient - this is suggested by a study published in September 2019 in Psychological Science.

University of Texas researchers asked 334 people to write a letter expressing gratitude to someone who did something nice for them. In the next step, the respondents were to guess how the recipient would feel, based on some questions. Then the researchers collaborated with the recipients to learn about their real responses.

Understanding the impact of a gesture (writing a letter of gratitude) can inspire people to do it more often. It is a great source of happiness for the recipient and giver.

So, take some time to write and send a well-deserved thank you. **This will be good for both of you.**

BE ACTIVE

Benefits such as mental stimulation and social engagement are associated with the hindrance of chronic diseases.

Good for health

Some studies link delayed retirement to better health and longevity. The study was conducted in 2016 on a group of about 3 thousand people, published in the Journal of Epidemiology and Community Health, suggesting that working for a year longer than the **standard age of retirement was associated with a 9-11% lower risk of death.**

According to data from the U.S. Bureau of Labor Statistics in 2017, those who were employed were:
32% of people aged 65 to 69,
19% of people aged 70 to 74 years.

It is estimated that in 2024, 36% of people aged 65 to 69 will be in the workforce – that is 22% more people in this age group than in 1994. These are good statistics for our health!

What should you do?

Work as long as possible!
Even if you are already retired, stay mentally, socially and physically active - just like in your professional life - it's good for your health.

- *Physical Stimulation* and problem resolution are good for maintaining your thinking skills
- *Social engagement* is linked to the hindrance of chronic diseases.
- *Remaining physically active*, even if it means only walking, can lead to better health as well as sharper thinking skills.

BRAIN TRAINING

A new study published on January 4, 2018 by the Journal of the American Geriatrics Society has shown that brain training can help people with mild cognitive impairment (MCI) who usually have memory impairment.

Researchers employed 145 adults diagnosed with MCI with an average age of 72 years. These people were divided into three groups.

I. The members of the first group had a two-hour brain training session in a week. The training focused on improving memory and learning how to better encode information, including the method of loci, i.e. associating images / situations with certain defined locations. They also practiced how to manage their attention better.

II. The members of the second group also took part in a two-hour training in a week. They were taught how to focus on the positive aspects of life, through dealing with stress and frustration.

III. The members of the third group did not take part in any program.

All participants underwent memory testing at the beginning and at the end of the study. The members of the first group received up to four times more points in the final test than the participants of the other groups. In addition, they maintained their improvement within six months of completing their training. Researchers speculated that it was because they used their training in everyday life.

More research is needed in this area, but the results suggest that stimulating the brain may be beneficial in improving memory, especially if done on a regular basis.

4 TRICKS TO IMPROVE YOUR MEMORY

Always be ahead of age-related changes in thinking skills. Make the most of your brain´s memory.

We all have moments of forgetting where we placed our keys or why we entered the room. This most likely reflects age-related changes in thinking skills.

„When it comes to the functioning of the brain, everyone deteriorates in all areas over time, except for vocabulary."

- says Dr. Joel Salinas, a neurologist specializing in behavioral neurology and neuropsychiatry in the Harvard-associated Massachusetts General Hospital.

How does memory work?

Memory consists of three processes:
1. Encoding
2. Storage
3. Recall

Many regions in the brain are involved in this process. For example, the cerebral cortex - the large outer layer of the brain - acquires new information as input from our senses. The amygdala marks information as worthy of storage. Nearby, the hippocampus holds memories. And the frontal lobes help us to consciously retrieve information.

There are noticeable changes in the brain from the time we reach 50 years-of-age. The chemical and structural processes that occur with age can slow down the speed of information processing, making it difficult to recall already known changes and words. Other factors may also exist.

„Working memory - a mental notebook that allows us to benefit from important information throughout the day - is prone to depression, anxiety and stress," explains Dr. Salinas, „Lack of sleep can affect the behavior and use of information by the brain."

What can I do to enhance memory?
Make the most of it. The following strategies can help:

1. Repeat out loud
Repetition increases the likelihood of saving information and retrieving it later.
„With each repetition, your brain has yet another way to encode information," explains Dr. Salinas, „The connections between brain cells are strengthened, similar to a burning trail in the forest. The more you follow the same trail, the easier it will be to go next time."

2. Make notes
Make a note of the people you need to call, things you need to do and meetings. *„We are much better at recognition than at recall,"* explains Dr. Salinas, *„Through recognition, such as reading a list, you have extra hooks or hints to help you find the information you are looking for."*

3. Associate old and new information.
Associate a person's name with something familiar. For example, if the person's name is Sandy, imagine that person on the beach, and when creating a shopping list, invent a story for it.
„Our brain is good at sequencing, and putting things into a story helps. The more ridiculous, the more memorable. For example, if your list is milk, eggs and bread, the story may be that you drink milk from Elvis over an egg sandwich" - suggests Dr. Salinas.

4. Split information into parts

„It is difficult to store a long number," says Dr. Salinas, *„However, it is easier to store smaller pieces into working memory".*

If you are trying to memorize a speech or a wedding toast, focus on one sentence or idea at a time, not on the whole speech all at once

When tricks do not help...

Forgetting something small from time to time is probably normal. It is not normal when changes in memory interfere with daily functioning. Dr. Salinas recommends talking to your doctor if you make more mistakes than usual at work; having difficulty paying bills; or having trouble completing tasks, cooking, sending emails or doing housework. **But don't panic.**

„There often is a temporary or reversible cause behind your memory slips. Once you take care of it, you can go back to your usual way of remembering", says Dr. Salinas.

EXERCISES

1. Match and place the given pairs of letters in the missing spaces so that they form the correct words.

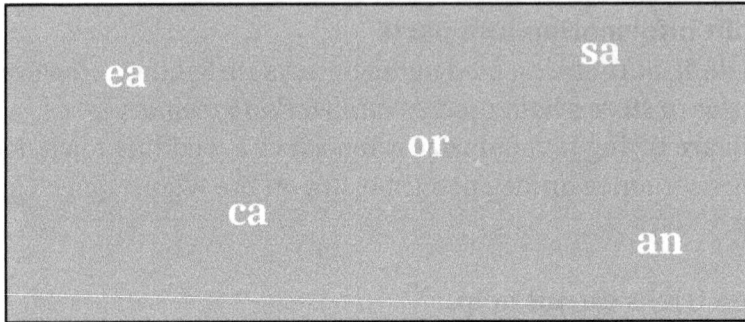

ea	sa
or	
ca	an

Words with missing letters	Space for your answers
- - thodontist	
- - nadi - -	
peli - - n	
co - - di - - t - -	
naus - -	
- - maritan	
- - dwich	
ar - -	
pl - -	
pi - - o	
hum - -	
harmoni - -	
- - - -	
vi - -	
- - mpling	

```
        se              uy
  pa
                    se
                           he
       ud
```

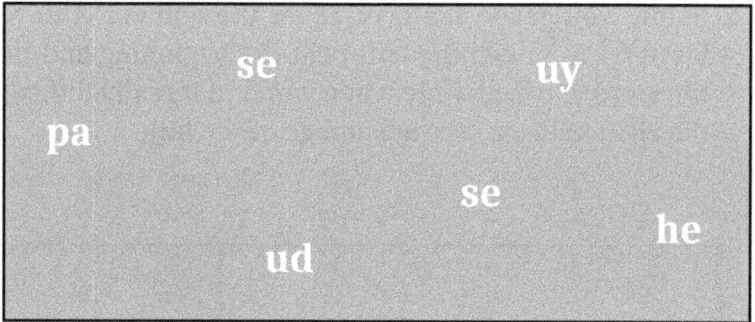

Words with missing letters	Space for your answers
b - -	
clo - -	
- - - - city	
- - licopter	
ab - - nces	
- - mochód	
- - ir	

Example:
- - mera is camera

2. Before you get to the task, cover the column with the hints. First, try to match the letters at the beginning and the end of the word yourself. Only when you find it really difficult to find the right answer, take advantage of the hint.

Words with missing letters	Space for your answers	Answers
- - welry b - -		wooden box
- rinte -		machine for printing
dre - -		home location
- - termel - -		a green fruit that looks like a ball
- oncer -		with an orchestra
- - intin -		in a museum
- ol -		in an egg
- ee - -		four on a car
- tar -		in the night sky

3. Intuicyjnie odpowiedz na poniższe pytania „prawda" lub „fałsz".

An elephant is bigger than a tiger.		true		false
Cherry juice is white like water.		true		false
Red beets prevent anemia.		true		false
All mushrooms are poisonous.		true		false
The capital of France is Paris.		true		false
An eagle is freer than a sparrow.		true		false
Turmeric has a yellow color.		true		false
A pillow is heavier than a blanket.		true		false
An elephant is bigger than an ostrich		true		false
Blueberries have the same taste as raspberries		true		false
Roses have thorns.		true		false
Sour cherry juice has the color of orange juice.		true		false
Palms grow as fast as spruces.		true		false
Aluminum foil can be placed in a microwave		true		false
Ontario is a city in the United States.		true		false
Vancouver is a city in Canada.		true		false

4. Try to find the answer to the questions below straight from your head and then write it in the designated space.

Questions	Space for your answers
How many minutes do 4 hours have?	
How many seconds do two and a half hours have?	
It will be five in the morning in eight hours. What time is it?	
How many days does each month have?	
How many weeks do we have in a year?	
It will be eight in the evening in twelve hours. What time is it?	
How many months do the seasons have?	

5. Find the mistakes in the given words, then write them correctly.

Incorrect word	Corrected word
diicsplnie	
ospt	
btotel	
virer	
tlephneoe	
rssciso	
richa	
ylowel	
ltfenep	
eprsu	
abckapck	
cntyrou	
tcyi	
obkos	
caepe	
upc	
yuttberfl	
pigniatn	
efcofe	
mgmaa	

6. Find and write words according to the instructions below.

List 5 cities for each letter, "K" and "L"

_____

_____

_____

_____

_____

List 5 cities for each letter, "S" and "P"

_____

_____

_____

_____

_____

List 5 plants for the letter "M"

_____

_____

_____

_____

_____

List 5 vegetables for the letter "O"

_____

_____

_____

_____

_____

7. Find and write letters that are in common for all words in the group:

Word Group	Space for your answers
dedication meditation medicine	
deduction reduction production	
baker bricklayer banker	
euthanasia Anastasia ambrosia	
area azalea	
larva diva Geneva	
mundane punctual punctuation	
juvenile rejuvenate	
margarine parkour art	
comedy Cody	
telephone gramophone saxophone	

Example:

chef, theft	ef

8. Make nine words from the scattered letter pairs

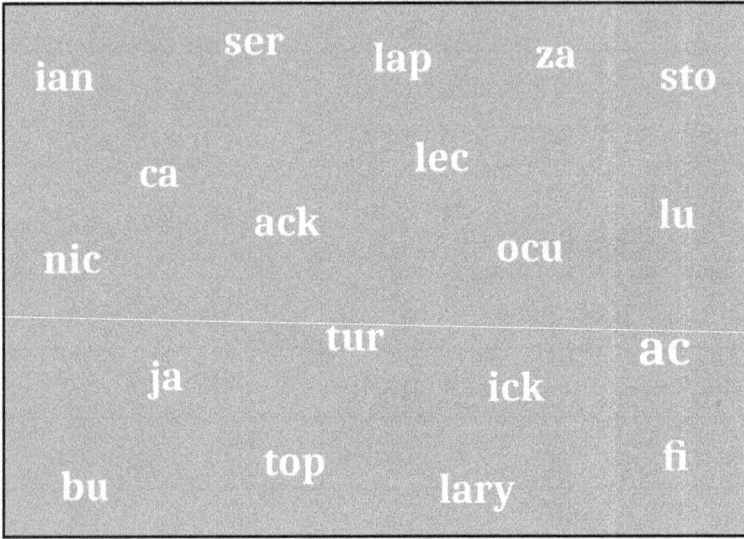

ian ser lap za sto

ca lec

ack lu

nic ocu

tur ac

ja ick

top fi

bu lary

_____

_____

_____

_____

_____

_____

_____

_____

9. Add the missing word to the sentence by finding it in the box

Canada   milk   books

fruitcake   parsley

Polański   London   fruits

Brussels   Joseph

wood

Warsaw

milk   Adams

Chopin

Phrases	Space for your answers
Furniture is 80% made of...	
A cow provides us with a white liquid called...	
Juice is made from...	
The European Union headquarters is located in....	
Butter is made from...	
The Polish capital is...	
In a library we read...	
The English capital is...	
The popular Polish composer born in Żelazowa Wola is...	
A popular baked good for Christmas is...	
An important biblical name is...	
An herb used for soups is...	
The famous Polish film director is Roman...	
The country that sits north to the USA is...	
A Canadian singer is Bryan..	

10. Fill out the missing letters in the words below.

Word	Hint	Space for your answers
s - - - e	shows up on your face when you are happy	
d - - - h	unbaked bread	
- - k -	mode of transport	
f - - - s - -	trees grow there	
m - - - - m -	you look at paintings and sculptures there	
- c - - r - - -	cold and sweet	
- o - - - - - e -	something black used in some cakes	
- r - e - - - -	the favorite drink of the Japanese	
b - - - s	in the library	
c - r	in a parking lot	

11. Complete the following words with the letters in the box and then add your own examples of words that have the same pairs of letters.

um	**na**	**tel**	
	ca		**sa**

Words with missing letters	Space for your answers
- - - ephone	
ho - - -	
- - - - tori - -	
mec - -	
for - -	
pas - - ge	
hye - -	
aquari - -	
asyl	
- - - ecommunication	
- - - egraph	
- - - evision	
- - r - - tion	
mo - - rchy	
doc - - ent	
cir - -	
a - - logy	
- - nd	
- - pture	

12. In the words below, underline the fruit with one line and underline the vegetables with two lines.

plum	tomato	orange	peas
radish	cauliflower		pear
beans	potatoes	cherries	spinach
apple	raspberry		blackberry
leek	celery	melon	mango
blueberries	cabbage	brussel sprout	onion

13. Write words from the box in alphabetic order, divided into rivers and flowers.

Rose	Vistula	Hyacinth	Volga	Violet
Seine	Danube	Sunflower	Thames	Ganges
Rhine	Main	Rhone	Amazon	
Nile	St. Lawrence	Tulip	Orchid	
Daisy	Poppy	Carnation		

River	Flowers

14. Sort the words into the table below.

> zebra   sparrow   hippopotamus   goldfinch
> elephant   owl   tiger   cheetah   jaguar
> peacock   eagle   chickadee   boar   deer
> crow   starling   woodpecker   parrot
> cormorant   pelican   squirrel   monkey
> panda   dog   bear   giraffe   kangaroo
> dudek   toucan   goat   roadrunner
> cat   cow   hummingbair   fox   pigeon

Birds	Other Animals

15. Sincerely answer the questions below and write down your answers.

What is my best and most beloved place, where I have time for myself?

_____

_____

_____

_____

What was my happiest day?

_____

_____

_____

_____

What was the most beautiful place that I have seen?

_____

_____

_____

_____

What do I like about winter?

_____

_____

_____

_____

What do I like about summer?

_____

_____

_____

_____

What do I like about autumn?

_____

_____

_____

_____

What do I like about spring?

_____

_____

_____

_____

What places would I like to? (list at least 10)

_____

_____

_____

_____

How much do I value the city / country that I live in?

_____

_____

_____

_____

What is my favorite meal? What do I like to cook?

_____

_____

_____

_____

What are my passions?

_____

_____

_____

_____

What am I excellent at, and what must I improve?

_____

_____

_____

_____

Do I have a favorite book? Which one?

_____

_____

_____

_____

What gives me happiness and peace?

_____

_____

_____

_____

What stresses me out and how do I deal with it?

_____

_____

_____

_____

How do I define respect? How much do I respect myself on a scale of 1-10?

_____

_____

_____

_____

How do I treat other people around me?

_____

_____

_____

_____

What are my biggest dreams? (list at least 3)

_____

_____

_____

_____

What would I like to do for my friends?

_____

_____

_____

_____

What would I like to learn?

_____

_____

_____

_____

What colors relax me?

_____

_____

_____

_____

Who motivates me and why?

_____

_____

_____

_____